Low Carb

Cookbook

(50 Mouthwatering Low Carb Recipes

For Rapid Weight Loss!)

2nd Edition

Athar Husain

INTRODUCTION

This book having **50** ultimate **mouthwatering Low-Carb** recipes. All the recipes are best in taste and required **minimum time** to **cook**. The Low-Carbohydrate Diet is very **beneficial** for **Weight Loss** and **reclaim energy**.

The recipes are very **yummy** and easy to cook. Reason, behind the popularity of **Low-Carb Diet** is that, it helps to reduce weight and also help to prevent **Diabetes**, **cardiovascular disease** and **high Blood Pressure.**

This Book contains **Delicious** Breakfast, Lunch, Dinner, Soups, Side Dishes, Salads and Snacks Recipes in **one pack**. So just discard your old boring recipes book and try this delicious **mouthwatering Low-Carb** recipes book today.

Table of Contents

Side Dishes:-

1. **Marvelous Mediterranean Vegetables.**
2. **Fast Italian Vegetable Skillet.**
3. **Skillet Fish with Spinach.**
4. **Grilled Zucchini with onions.**
5. **Pleasing Peas and Asparagus.**
6. **Spicy Grilled Eggplant.**
7. **Tangy Italian Green Beans.**
8. **Creamy Cheddar Broccoli.**

Salads:-

1. **Easy Caesar Salad.**
2. **Balsamic Vegetable Salad.**
3. **Maple Salad Dressing.**
4. **Kansas Cucumber Salad.**
5. **Vanilla Fruit Salad.**
6. **Quick Avocado Tomato Salad.**
7. **Mint Watermelon Salad.**
8. **Herbed Tuna Salad.**

Soups:-

1. **Sausage Pizza Soup.**
2. **Hearty Beef Soup.**
3. **Homemade Creamy Tomato Soup.**
4. **Marvelous Mushroom Soup.**
5. **Smooth Carrot Soup.**
6. **Reuben Soup.**
7. **Cream of Cauliflower Soup.**

Snacks:-

1. Chocolate Pro Cake.
2. Mini Cheeseburger Pies.
3. Spinach Loaf.
4. Cheese Spread.
5. Spinach Egg Muffins.
6. Herbed Tortilla Chips.
7. Tuna Bites.
8. Egg Muffins with Turkey Sausage.

1. Skillet-Baked Eggs with Spinach, Chili Oil and Yogurt.

Ingredients:-

- 2/3 cup Greek-style yogurt, plain
- 1/2garlic clove
- Kosher salt
- 2 tsp. olive oil
- 2 tsp. unsalted butter
- 2 tsp. chopped scallion (pale green and white parts only)
- 3 tsp. chopped leek (pale green and white parts only)
- 10 cups fresh spinach (10 ounces)
- 3/2 tsp. fresh lemon juice
- 4 large eggs
- A pinch of paprika and 1/4 tsp. crushed red pepper flakes or 1/4 teaspoon Kirmizi biber.
- 1 tsp. chopped fresh oregano.

Instructions:-

1. Take a small bowl and mix garlic with yogurt and a pinch of salt in it.
2. Heat up oven to 300°. Dissolve 1 full tablespoon butter with oil in a large heavy skillet over medium heat Add some leek and scallion; decrease heat to low. Cook about 10 minutes, until it become soft. Put on some spinach and lemon juice with salt. Again raise heat to high; cook, turn repeatedly, until properly cooked, it takes 4-5 minutes.
3. Take spinach mixture to a big skillet. Divide spinach mixture equally between skillets, if you are using 2 smaller skillets. Make 4 deep cavities in center of spinach in larger skillet or 2 cavities in each small skillet. Break 1 egg into each cavity, taking care to keep yolks intact. Bake egg whites, 10-15 minutes.
4. Dissolve remaining 1 tablespoon butter in a small skillet over low heat. Put kirmizi biber and a pinch of salt and prepare until butter starts to foam and browned bits form at bottom of pan it takes 1-2 minutes. Put oregano and cook for 30 seconds. Separate garlic halves from yogurt. Spoon yogurt over spinach and eggs. Dribble with spiced butter.

2. Egg Crust Breakfast Pizza with Olives, Pepperoni, Tomatoes and Mozzarella.

Ingredients:-

- 1-2 tsp. olive oil (depending on the size of your pan).
- 2 Eggs, beaten properly
- 4-5 small tomatoes, slice the tomatoes as thinly as possible
- 6 slices of turkey pepperoni, chop in half to make half-moon pieces
- 1 oz. low-fat mozzarella, slice into small cubes
- Spike seasoning according to taste (about 1/2 teaspoon.)
- Dry oregano, according to taste (about 1/4 teaspoon.)

Instructions:-

1. Heat up broiler in oven or small toaster oven. Break eggs into a small pot and mix them well. Thinly Sliced olives and tomatoes, chopped pepperoni into 2 halves, and slice mozzarella into small cubes.
2. Put small amount of olive oil to the omelet frying pan and heat over medium heat until the pan is get hot nearly 1 minute. Mixed the eggs with spike seasoning and oregano, cook about 2 minutes or until eggs are properly cooked.
3. Drizzle on half each of the tomatoes, mozzarella, pepperoni and olives proceeded by a second layer with half of each. (Make ensure there should be plenty of cheese on the top layer.) Now cover up the pan and cook until the cheese is starting to dissolve and eggs are well cook, nearly 3 minutes.
4. Put pan under the broil and bake until the cheese is melted and the upper part is starting to brown, about 2-3 minutes with oven broiler and serve hot.

3. Baby Kale, Egg Bake and Mozzarella.

Ingredients:-

- 5 oz. mixed baby kale or chopped kale leaves
- 1-2 tsp. olive oil (depending on size of your pan)
- 3/2 cup mozzarella cheese (Low-Fat)
- 1/3 cup green onion slice as thin as possible
- 8 eggs
- 1 tsp. Spike Seasoning (You may choose any seasoning blend that tastes good with eggs instead of Spike.)
- fresh ground black pepper and salt according to taste

Instructions:-

1. Heat up the oven to 190C. Sprinkle an 8 &1/2 inch by 12 inch glass or crockery pot dish with olive oil.
2. Heat up the oil in a large skillet, mix the kale all at once, and stir until the kale is wither, nearly 1 minute for baby kale and 2-3 minutes for chopped kale. Fetch the kale to the crockery pot dish, in the way that all the bottom of the dish is covered. Make the layer of thinly sliced onions and mozzarella cheese on top of the kale.
3. Mix the Eggs with Spike Seasoning, fresh ground pepper and salt according to taste. (I use few grinds of pepper and a small pinch of salt) Splash the egg mixture over the kale and cheese combination, and then use a spoon to gently mix so the eggs, kale and cheese, are mixed properly.
4. Bake the mixture about 30-35 minutes until the mixture is starting to lightly brown. Now cools the dish about 5 minutes before cutting. Serve hot. This is tastier with light sour-cream. It will be tastier with little Green Tabasco Sauce dribble on the top.

4. Mini- Smoked Salmon Frittatas.

Ingredients:-

- 1 tsp. extra virgin oil
- 1/4 cup sliced onion
- 1/2 tsp. salt
- 1/8 tsp. pepper
- 4 oz. smoked salmon, cut into 1/4 inch slices
- 6 large eggs
- 8 large eggs white
- 3 tsp. 1% milk
- 3 oz. 1/3 less fat cream cheese
- 2 tsp. scallions, slice as thin as possible, for garnish

Instructions:-

1. Heat up oven to 325°. Heat oil in a non-stick large frying pan. Roast onion 2–3 minutes, add pepper, salmon and salt to taste. Remove from stove and let cool the mixture.
2. Mix the next 4 ingredients (through milk) in a pot. Mix in the cream cheese. Lightly coat 6 ramekins with cooking sprinkle. Add 2 tsp. of salmon mixture to every ramekin. Pour 3/4 cup egg mixture into every ramekin.
3. Put ramekins on baking sheet; bake 25 minutes or until a wooden pick inserted in center comes out clean. Then garnish.

5. Migas, My Way Recipe.

Ingredients:-

- 1/4 cup onion, cut into pieces
- 1/4 thinly sliced green pepper
- Drizzle 1 tsp. bacon or canola oil
- 4 Eggs
- 1 tsp. water
- 1 tsp. salsa
- 1/2 cup squashed tortilla chips
- Divided 1/2 cup finely sliced cheddar cheese
- Thinly sliced green onions, additional warm flour tortillas and salsa

Instructions:-

1. In a large frying pan, fry onion and green pepper drizzle until tender. In a small pot, beat the eggs, salsa and water. Add to frying pan, cook and mix them properly. Stir in tortilla chips and 1/4 cup cheese.
2. Splash with remaining cheese. Serve with tortillas, salsa and green onions.

Ingredients:-

- 1/2 lb. Mexican chorizo
- 1/2 small onion. Thinly sliced
- 2 garlic cloves, chopped
- 6 Eggs
- 1/4 cup whole milk
- 1/2 cup minced mozzarella cheese
- Fresh parsley, minced
- 3 bell peppers, tops cut and seeded
- Pepper and salt according to taste

Instructions:-

1. Heat up the oven to 350°F.
2. Bake chorizo in a large frying pan until it starts to brown.
3. Mix onion and garlic well. Bake about 3 minutes.
4. In a pot, mix beaten eggs, cheese, milk, parsley, pepper and salt.
5. Add chorizo to the pot and blend well.
6. Gush mixture in the bell peppers and place them in a shallow baking dish.
7. Bake for 35-40 minutes or until the eggs are thoroughly baked.

7. Easy Mushroom Quiche.

Ingredients:-

- 300g (11 ounce) freshly chopped mushroom
- 1 shallot, properly chopped
- 50g (2 ounce) butter
- 4 tsp. dried breadcrumbs
- 2 tsp. grated parmesan cheese
- 1/4 tsp. salt
- 1/4 tsp. fresh black pepper
- 100g (4 ounce) thinly sliced cheddar cheese
- 1 (200g) soft tub cream cheese
- 4 Eggs
- 1 dash tabasco sauce
- 150g (5 ounce) cooked bacon, diced
- Sliced fresh parsley to garnish

Instructions:-

1. Heat up oven to 190 degree C
2. Take a medium frying pan, fry mushrooms and onion in butter, about 5 minutes. Mix in the breadcrumbs, pepper, parmesan and salt according to taste.
3. Butter the bottom end sides of a 10 inch pie pan. Squeeze mushroom mixture into pan equally on bottom end side. Sprinkle shredded cheese over the mushroom.
4. In a blender, mix together Tabasco sauce, cream cheese and eggs. Stir in chopped bacon. Spill over the cheese and mushroom and bake about 30 minutes. Serve with freshly sliced parsley.

8. Mushroom Scrambled Eggs.

Ingredients:-

- 1/2 cup chopped fresh mushrooms
- 1/4 cup slice as thin as possible green onions
- 1 tsp. cooking oil
- 1 8 oz. container chilled iced egg product, thawed, or 4 eggs mixed properly
- 1/4 cup milk (Fat-Free)
- 1/8 tsp. fresh ground black pepper
- 1/2 cup finely chopped low-fat cheddar cheese (2 oz.) or blue cheese (2 oz.) or1/4 cup crushed feta
- 1 thinly sliced bacon, crunchy cooked and crushed
- 8 cherry tomatoes or grapes, cut into two halves

Instructions:-

1. A large unheated, nonstick skillet, coat up with nonstick cooking spray. Heat up skillet over medium heat. Add green onions and mushrooms. Mix in oil and cook about 6 minutes or until vegetables are well cooked.
2. Take a proper mixture of milk, egg and pepper in a medium bowl. Pour egg mixture into skillet. Cook, without stirring, until the mixture is well cook on the bottom and around edge. Using a large spoon, lift and fold partially cooked egg mixture so uncooked portion flows below.
3. Drizzle with bacon and cheese. Carry on cooking over medium heat about 2 to 3 minutes or until egg mixture is properly cooked. Remove from heat instantly. (Be aware not to overcook the egg mixture).
4. Serve with tomatoes.

9. Pick-Me-Up Bars.

Ingredients:-

- Non-Stick cooking spray
- 3 tsp. honey
- 1/4 cup fresh orange juice
- 2 cup fresh lemon juice
- 18-oz. package dates, chopped
- 2 1/2 cups whole wheat flour
- 1/2 tsp. baking soda
- 1/4 tsp. baking powder
- 1/4 cup unsweetened apple sauce
- 3 tsp. pure maple syrup
- 1 tsp. canola or cooking oil

Instructions:-

1. Heat up oven to 176 degrees Celsius. Take a 13x9x2-inch baking pan with foil. Set a foil lightly coated with cooking spray aside on baking pan. Mix the orange juice, honey and fresh lemon juice in a small bowl. Mix in the dates.
2. Mix the soda, baking powder and flour in a large pot. In a second mixing pot, mix egg whites, syrup, oil and apple sauce. Now add flour mixture to apple sauce mixture. Beat with an electric mixer until the mixture will be thoroughly crumble.

Lunch Recipes:-

1. Garlic Chicken

Ingredients:-

- 1/4 cup olive oil
- 1/4 Cup Parmesan Cheese, shredded
- 2 Cloves Garlic, minced
- 4, Chicken Breast Halves, boneless
- 1/4Cup Bread Crumbs, Italian-Seasoned

Instructions:-

1. Heat up oven to 220 degrees C.
2. Heat garlic and olive oil in a small skillet over medium heat until warmed for 1-2 minutes. Carry oil and garlic to a shallow pot.
3. Mix Parmesan cheese and bread crumbs in a separate shallow pot.
4. Dip chicken breasts in the garlic-olive oil mixture using forceps; shift to bread crumb mixture and turn to evenly coat. Shift coated chicken to a shallow baking dish.
5. Bake in the heated oven about 35 minutes. An immediate-read thermometer place into the center of dish. It should read at least 74 degrees C.

2. Spinach Stuffed Chicken Breast.

Ingredients:-

- 1 (10 oz.) fresh spinach leaves
- 4 chicken breast halves, boneless
- 1/2 cup sour cream
- 1 inch fresh ground black pepper
- 1/2 cup pepper jack cheese, shredded
- 8 slices of bacon
- 4 cloves garlic, chopped

Instructions:-

1. Heat up the oven to 190 degree c.
2. Put spinach in a large glass pot, and microwave for 3 minutes. Mix garlic and pepper jack cheese in sour cream.
3. On a clean surface put the chicken breasts, and brush the spinach mixture onto each side. First roll up chicken to enclose the spinach, then cover each chicken breast with two pieces of bacon. Protected with toothpicks, and place in a shallow baking dish.
4. Uncovered the dish and bake for 30 minutes in the microwave oven, then raise heat to 260 degree c, for an additional 7 minutes to brown the bacon.

3. Blackened Chicken.

Ingredients:-

- 1/2 tsp. paprika
- 1/4 tsp. dried thyme
- 1/8 tsp. salt
- 1/8 tsp. fresh ground white pepper
- 1/4 tsp. cayenne pepper
- 1/8 tsp. fresh onion powder
- 1/4 tsp. fresh ground cumin
- 2 chicken breast halves, boneless

Instructions:-

1. Heat up oven to 175 degree C. Gently coat the baking sheet. Heat a non-stick skillet over high temperature for 5 minutes.
2. Combine together cayenne, salt, paprika, thyme, white pepper, cumin and onion powder. Drizzle oil into the chicken breasts with cooking spray on both sides, then coat to toss the chicken breasts with the spice mixture.
3. Put the chicken in the hot skillet and cook for 2 minute. Turn the chicken and cook for 2 minutes on another side. Take the prepared baking sheet and put the breasts on it.
4. Bake in the heated microwave oven about 5 minutes.

4. Smoky Grilled Chicken with Zucchini Ramen Noodles.

Ingredients:-

For the Grilled Chicken

- 1/4 tsp. cayenne pepper
- 1 tsp. smoked paprika
- 1 tsp. chili powder
- 1/2 tsp. fresh garlic powder
- 1/2 tsp. fresh ground coriander
- 1/2 tsp. ground cumin
- 1/4 tsp. kosher salt to taste
- 1 tbsp. olive oil
- 1 pound chicken thighs (6), boneless

For the Ramen

- 2 small zucchini
- 1/4 tsp. cayenne pepper
- 1 tsp. smoked paprika
- 1 tsp. chili powder
- 1/2 tsp. fresh garlic powder
- 1/2 tsp. fresh ground coriander
- 1/2 tsp. fresh ground cumin
- 1/4 tsp. kosher salt to taste
- 1 tbsp. fresh coconut oil
- 1/2 cup red sweet peppers, sliced
- 1/2 cup fresh onions, thinly sliced
- 3 cups mixed raw vegetables
- 8 cups chicken stock

Instructions:-

1. Take two small mixing pot, place them side by side and in each pot, put 1/4 tsp. cayenne pepper, 1 tsp. chili powder, 1 tsp. smoked paprika, 1/2 tsp. fresh garlic powder, 1/2 tsp. fresh ground coriander, 1/2 tsp. fresh ground cumin, 1/4 tsp. kosher salt to taste.
2. Put the chicken in a glass mixing pot and mix all the mixture of spices in mixing pot, add 1 Tbsp. of olive oil. Keep the chicken to marinate for 1 hour.
3. Prepare long noodles from the zucchini using a spiralizer. Put aside.

4. Heat up the grate to high. Place the chicken on the grate, remove the marinade. Grill the Chicken for 5 minutes on one side and 4 minutes on another side. Allow the prepared chicken to sit for 5 minute and then cut into slices (lengthwise) 6 or 7 pieces. Place aside.
5. Keep the chicken stock to a boil in a large bowl.
6. While the chicken stock is reach to a boil, heat up 1 tbsp. of coconut oil in a large skillet over high heat. Mix the vegetables and the second pot of spices and fry for 2 minutes. Put the vegetables on a plate to prevent over cooking and put aside.
7. Mix the zucchini "ramen" to the boiling chicken stock and stop the supply of heat.
8. Pour the soup mixture into 5 bowls and dribble with the grilled chicken and seasoned vegetables.
9. Serve with sriracha and eat with chopsticks and a spoon.

5. Cauliflower Pizza Crust Recipe.

Ingredients:-

- 1 small head of cauliflower, removed leaves and stems
- 1 tsp. basil
- 1 tsp. fresh oregano
- 1 tsp. fresh parsley
- 1 tsp. salt
- 1/2 cup Mozzarella
- 2 eggs
- Cornmeal, to dust the pizza stone

For Pizza

- 1 jug pizza sauce
- 1/2 cup sheep milk cheese
- 7-9 basil leaves

Instructions:-

1. Heat up the oven to 176 degree C.
2. Cut the cauliflower florets into large pieces. Now in the food processor pulse the cauliflower until it look like a fine grain, like rice. Take a large pot and pour the cauliflower into pot. Mix salt and herbs, then eggs and cheese.
3. Then disperse cornmeal all over a pizza stone. Keep the cauliflower mixture on the middle of the stone and by using your hands to press it into a circle about 1/4 inch thick.
4. Bake for 20 minutes at 176 degree C then an additional 12 minutes at 200 degree C. Crust will be done when it became golden brown in color.
5. Take out crust from oven. Increase the oven temperature to 232 degrees C. Mix pizza sauce, cheese and then bake again for 7 minutes or until cheese on top is dissolved.

Dinner Recipes:-

1. Tuscan Chicken Recipe.

Ingredients:-

- 4 chicken breast halves (boneless, skinless)
- 1/2 tsp. salt
- 1/2 tsp. pepper
- 2 thinly sliced garlic cloves
- 2 tsp. rosemary, dried and crumpled
- 1/2 tsp. rubbed sage
- 1/2 tsp. thyme, dried
- 2 tbsp. olive oil

Instructions:-

1. Sliced the chicken to 1/2 inch thickness pieces and drizzle with pepper and salt to taste.
2. Take a large frying pan, cook and mix the garlic, sage, rosemary and thyme in oil for 2 minute over medium heat. Mix chicken and cook for 7-8 minutes on each side or until chicken cooked well.

2. Fontina-Fruit Chicken Breast.

Ingredients:-

- 1/3 cup olive oil
- 3 tbsp. cider vinegar
- 2 tbsp. red wine vinegar
- 2 tsp. honey
- 1 tsp. Dijon mustard
- 1/2 tsp. fresh ground mustard
- 8 chicken breast halves, boneless
- 1 large tart apple, shredded and peeled
- 1 tsp. butter
- 1/2 cup fontina cheese, chopped
- 1/2 cherries, thinly sliced and dried
- 1/2 tsp. salt
- 1/2 tsp. pepper

Instructions:-

1. Mix the first 6 ingredients into large disposable poly bag. Cut a cavity in each chicken breast half and put in the bag. Seal and coat fully with the mixture, refrigerate for 5 minutes.
2. Take a small nonstick frying pan and fry apple in butter until it fried well. Transfer to a small pot. Mix pepper, cherries and salt in the cheese. Filter chicken from marinade then mix with apple mixture. Protected with soaked toothpicks.
3. Take a paper towel and wet with cooking oil, by using long handed tongs, finely coat the grate rack. Cover the chicken and grill over medium heat on each side or until the temperature reaches to 170 degree C. Remove toothpicks.

3. Herbed Lemon Pork Chops.

Ingredients:-

- 1 tsp. salt-free garlic seasoning blend
- 1/2 tsp. basil, dried
- 1/2 tsp. oregano, dried
- 1/2 tsp. fresh parsley, thinly sliced
- 1/4 tsp. salt
- 1/4 tsp. rosemary crumpled and dried
- 2 bone-in pork loin chop (6 oz. each)
- 1 tsp. olive oil
- 1 garlic clove, chopped
- 1 tbsp. fresh lemon juice

Instructions:-

1. Take a small pot and mix first six ingredients. Coat over both sides of pork chops. Take a large nonstick frying pan. Heat garlic and oil over medium-high heat. Add pork chops, cook for 5 minutes on each side.
2. Take away from heat and sprinkle with lemon juice. Cover and keep aside for 3 minutes before serving.

4. Creole Pork Chops.

Ingredients:-

- 1/2 tsp. salt
- 1/2 tsp. basil, dried
- 1/2 tsp. paprika
- 1/2 tsp. ground pepper
- 1/4 tsp. ground cumin
- 1/8 to 1/4 fresh cayenne pepper
- 4 pork loin chops, boneless
- 2 tbsp. canola oil
- 1 tin can (8 oz.) tomato sauce
- 1/2 cup onion, sliced
- 1/2 cup green pepper, sliced
- 1/4 cup fresh celery, chopped
- 1 tbsp. Worcestershire sauce
- 1/2 tsp. garlic, shredded

Instructions:-

1. Take a small pot, mix first six ingredients and coat over both sides of pork.
2. Take a large frying pan and cook loin chips in oil over medium heat about 3 minutes on each sides or until the color of chops changes to light brown, then filter. Combine the remaining ingredients. Cover and cook for 5 minutes longer or until the temperature of thermometer reaches 145 degree. Keep aside for 5 minutes before serving.

5. Brown sugar-glazed salmon.

Ingredients:-

- 1 salmon fillet (1 lb.)
- 1/4 tsp. salt
- 1/4 tsp. ground pepper
- 3 tbsp. brown sugar
- 1 tbsp. soy sauce (low-sodium)
- 4 tsp. Dijon mustard
- 1 tsp. rice vinegar

Instructions:-

1. Sliced the salmon widthwise into four pieces. Take a foil lined baking pan, sized 15-in. x 10-in. x 1-in. and place the salmon in it. Drizzle with pepper and salt. Uncovered and bake for 10 minutes at 425 degree.
2. At the same time take a small saucepan and mix soy sauce, brown sugar, vinegar and mustard. Let the mixture to boil. Coat evenly over salmon and grill 6 inch from the heat for 2 minutes or until the salmon properly grilled.

Side Dishes:-

1. Marvelous Mediterranean Vegetables.

Ingredients:-

- 3 thinly sliced large fresh Portobello mushrooms
- 1 each thinly sliced medium sweet red, yellow and orange peppers
- 1 medium thinly sliced zucchini
- Cut 10 fresh asparagus spears into 2 inch lengths
- 1 thinly sliced small onion, separated into rings
- 3/4 cup fresh grape tomatoes
- Half cup fresh sugar snap peas
- Half cup fresh broccoli florets
- Half cup pitted Greek olives
- 1 bottle (14 oz.) Greek vinaigrette
- Half cup crumpled feta cheese

Instructions:-

1. Take a large plastic bag, mix the zucchini, mushrooms and peppers. Combine the asparagus, peas, tomatoes, onions, broccoli and olives. Drizzle vinaigrette into the bag then seal bag and stir them to evenly coat in the bag. Store at the low temperature for at least half an hour.
2. Remove marinade and put all the vegetables to a grill basket. Just uncovered and grilled over medium heat for 8-10 minutes and stir regularly. Serve and trickle with cheese.

2. Fast Italian Vegetable Skillet.

Ingredients:-

- 1 onion cut into two halved
- 1 medium sweet red pepper, minced
- 1 tbsp. olive oil
- 3 thinly sliced medium zucchini
- 1 fresh garlic clove, shredded
- 1-1/2 cups icy corn, defrosted
- 1 large fresh tomato, sliced
- 2 tsp. fresh basil, shredded
- 1/2 tsp. salt
- 1/2 tsp. Italian seasoning
- 1/4 cup shredded fresh parmesan cheese

Instructions:-

1. Take a large non-stick frying pan, fry red pepper and onion in oil for 3 minutes. Mix zucchini and fry for 4-5 minutes or until vegetables are become crispy. Mix garlic, cook about 2 minutes.
2. Mix in the basil, tomato, corn, Italian seasoning and salt to taste then cook and stir until heated properly. Drizzle with cheese. Serve instantly.

3. Skillet Fish with Spinach.

Ingredients:-

- 4 orange roughy fillets (4 oz. each)
- 1-1/2 tsp. seafood seasoning
- 2 tbsp. olive oil
- 2 tbsp. butter
- 1 cup fresh mushrooms, chopped
- 1 package (10 oz.) icy minced spinach, defrosted and drain
- 1/2 cup chicken broth
- Pepper and salt

Instructions:-

1. Drizzle fillets with seafood seasoning. Take a large skillet and cook fillets in oil and butter over medium-low heat for 4 minutes on each sides. Take out and heat up.
2. Put the mushrooms to the skillet, uncovered and cook for 3-4 minutes or until mushrooms cooked properly. Mix spinach and broth and cook for 4-5 minutes or until spinach is heated fully. Season with pepper and salt. Serve with fish.

4. Grilled zucchini with onions.

Ingredients:-

- 6 small fresh zucchini, cut into halved lengthwise
- 4 tsp. olive oil
- 2 thinly sliced fresh green onions
- 2 tbsp. fresh lemon juice
- 1/2 tsp. salt
- 1/8 tsp. red pepper flakes, crushed

Instructions:-

1. Drizzle zucchini with 2 tsp. oil. Grill and covered, over medium heat for 10 minutes or until cooked properly, turn only once.
2. Put in the large pot. Combine the fresh lemon juice, green onions, pepper flakes, salt, lemon and remaining oil and shake them up in the pot.

5. Pleasing Peas and Asparagus.

Ingredients:-

- 1/2 cup water
- 2 packages (10 oz. each) icy peas
- 3/4 lbs. fresh asparagus, chopped into 1-inch pieces
- 3 tbsp. butter
- 1 tbsp. fresh parsley, minced
- 3/4 tsp. garlic salt
- Small pinch of pepper

Instructions:-

1. Bring water to boil in the large saucepan. Combine butter, asparagus, peas, parsley, garlic salt and pepper. Combine back to boil.
2. Decrease heat, cover and cook until asparagus become crispy, for approx.10 minutes. Filter and serve at once.

6. Spicy Grilled Eggplant.

Ingredients:-

- 2 1/2-inch sliced small eggplant
- 1/4 cup olive oil
- 2 tbsp. fresh lime juice
- 1 tbsp. Cajun seasoning

Instructions:-

1. Whisk eggplant slices with oil on both sides. Drizzle with fresh lime juice and mix with Cajun seasoning. Let wait for 5 minutes.
2. Cover the eggplant over medium heat for 4-5 minutes on each side or until cooked properly.

7. Tangy Italian Green Beans.

Ingredients:-

- 1/2 lbs. fresh or icy cut green beans
- 2 tbsp. water
- 2-1/4 tsp. shredded parmesan cheese
- 2-1/4 tsp. seasoned bread crumbs
- 1/4 tsp. garlic salt
- 1/8 tsp. pepper
- 1-1/2 tsp. olive oil

Instructions:-

1. Put water and beans in a microwave safe dish. Cover and turn on microwave for 5 minutes or till it turns to crispy.
2. Take a small pot, combine the bread, crumbs, cheese, pepper and garlic salt. Filter the beans and drizzle with olive oil. Trickle with cheese mixture and shake them up in the bowl.

8. Creamy Cheddar Broccoli.

Ingredients:-

- 3 cups fresh broccoli florets
- 2 tbsp. water
- 3 tbsp. soft cream cheese
- 2 tbsp. 2% milk
- 1-1/2 tsp. salad dressing mix
- 2 tbsp. cheddar cheese, chopped

Instructions:-

1. Put the water and broccoli in the 1-qt microwave-safe dish. Cover and turn on microwave for 3 minutes or until it becomes crispy. Take a small bowl, mix the cream cheese, milk and salad dressing mix.
2. Filter broccoli and coming back to dish. Place cream cheese mixture and drizzle with cheddar cheese. Cover and microwave at 60% power about 2 minutes or until heated fully and cheese is melted.

Salads:-

1. Easy Caesar Salad.

Ingredients:-

- 1/4 cup shredded parmesan cheese
- 1/4 full cup mayonnaise
- 2 tbsp. milk
- 1 tbsp. fresh lemon juice
- 1 tbsp. Dijon-mayonnaise blend
- 1 garlic clove, shredded
- Dash cayenne pepper
- 1 bunch romaine, torn
- Salad croutons

Instructions:-

1. In a small mixing pot, mix the first seven ingredients. Put down romaine in a large mixing pot. Drizzle with dressing and dish up with salad croutons.

2. Balsamic Vegetable Salad.

Ingredients:-

- 3 large tomatoes, cut into equally halved pieces
- 3 medium cucumbers thinly sliced halved and peeled
- 1/2 cup fresh olive oil
- 1/4 cup fresh balsamic vinegar
- 3 tbsp. water
- 1 packet Italian salad dressing mix.

Instructions:-

1. In a salad pot, mix cucumbers and tomatoes. In a small pot, mix the vinegar, water, oil and dressing mix. Drizzle over vegetables and shake them up in the bowl.

3. Maple Salad Dressing.

Ingredients:-

- 7 tbsp. maple syrup
- 1/4 cup fresh cider vinegar
- 1/4 cup fresh ketchup
- 3 tbsp. + 1 tsp. canola oil
- 2 tbsp. water
- 1/2 tsp. prepared horse radish
- 1/4 tsp. salt to taste
- 1/8 tsp. celery salt according to taste

Instructions:-

1. In a small mixing pot, mix all the ingredients. Till servings refrigerate and cover the dish.

4. Kansas Cucumber Salad.

Ingredients:-

- 1 cup miracle whip
- 1/4 cup sugar
- 4 tsp. fresh cider vinegar
- 1/2 tsp. dill weed
- 1/2 tsp. salt to taste
- 4 medium cucumbers, chopped and peeled
- 3 green onions, sliced

Instructions:-

1. In a large mixing pot, add sugar, dill, vinegar, salt miracle whip mix well. Mix properly cucumbers and onions together. Cover and refrigerate for min 1 hour.

5. Vanilla Fruit Salad.

Ingredients:-

- 5 tin cans (20 oz. each) plus 1 tin can (8 oz.) pineapple nugget
- 4 packages (5.1 oz. each) instant vanilla pudding mix
- 8 tin cans (15 oz. each) mandarin oranges, drained
- 10 medium fresh red apples, minced

Instructions:-

1. Drain pineapple juice from pineapple, keep the pineapple aside. Mix enough water to juice to make 6 cups.
2. Take a very large bowl and whip juice mixture and pudding mix for two minutes. Let stand for 2 minutes. Mix in the reserved pineapple, oranges and apples. Refrigerate until the mixture become chilled.

6. Quick Avocado Tomato Salad.

Ingredients:-

- 2-1/2 cups torn mixed salad greens
- 1/2 cup cherry tomatoes
- 1 medium, properly peeled and thinly sliced, ripe avocado
- 1/4 cup real bacon bits
- 2 tbsp. canola oil
- 1 tbsp. fresh cider vinegar
- 1/2 tsp. salt to taste

Instructions:-

1. Take four salad plates divide the avocado, greens and tomatoes among four salad plates the trickle with bacon. Take a small bowl and whip the remaining ingredients. Drizzle over salad.

7. Mint Watermelon Salad.

Ingredients:-

- 1 tbsp. fresh lemon juice
- 1 tbsp. olive oil
- 2 tsp. sugar to taste
- 6 cups fresh watermelon, seedless and cut into cubes.
- 2 tbsp. fresh mint, minced
- Fresh lemon wedges

Instructions:-

1. Take a small bowl and mix the olive oil, sugar and fresh lemon juice. Take a large bowl, mix seedless watermelon and minced mint. Drizzle with fresh lemon juice mixture, shake them up in the bowl. Garnish with fresh lemon wedges.

8. Herbed Tuna Salad.

Ingredients:-

- 1 tin can (6 oz.) light water-packed flaked tuna, drained
- 2 tbsp. finely sliced red onion
- 1 tsp. fresh parsley, shredded
- 1-1/2 tsp. dill weed
- 1/8 tsp. garlic salt to taste
- 1/8 tsp. dried thyme
- 1/8 tsp. ground pepper
- Small pinch of cayenne pepper
- 2 tbsp. mayonnaise (Fat-Free)
- 1 tbsp. sour cream (Low-Fat)
- 3 cups green salads, spring mix
- Chop 1 medium tomato into wedges

Instructions:-

1. Take a small dish pot, mix the first 8 ingredients then mix sour cream and mayonnaise and pour into the tuna mixture.
2. Take two plates and divide the salad greens between them. Sprinkle with tomato wedges and tuna mixture.

Soups:-

1. Sausage pizza Soup.

Ingredients:-

- 1/2 lbs. Italian turkey sausage
- 1 medium zucchini, thinly sliced
- 1 cup finely chopped fresh mushrooms
- 1 small onion, thinly sliced
- 1 container (14-1/2 oz.) no-salt-added chopped tomatoes
- 1 cup water
- 1 cup reduced-sodium chicken broth
- 1 tsp. dried basil
- 1/4 tsp. fresh pepper
- Shredded fresh basil; and crumpled red pepper flakes

Instructions:-

1. In a large skillet, cook the zucchini, mushrooms, onion and sausage over medium-low heat until meat is no longer pink; drain. Add the fresh pepper, water, broth, dried basil and tomatoes. Fetch to boil. Lower the heat; simmer, open, for 15 minutes. Drizzle with fresh basil and pepper flakes.

2. Hearty Beef Soup.

Ingredients:-

- 4 pounds beef top sirloin steak, minced into 1/2 inches cubes
- 4 cup thinly sliced onions
- 1/4 cup butter
- 4 quarts hot water
- 4 cups sliced carrots
- 4 cups cubed potatoes, peeled
- 2 cups thinly sliced cabbage
- 1 cup thinly sliced celery
- 1 large green pepper, thinly sliced
- 8 tsp. beef bouillon granules
- 1 tsp. seasoned salt to taste
- 1 tsp. dried basil
- 1 tsp. fresh pepper
- 4 bay leaves
- 6 cups fresh tomato juice

Instructions:-

1. Take brown beef and onion in butter in batches, in two Dutch ovens and drain. Add the water, seasonings and vegetables, bring to boil. Turn down the heat; cover and cook gently for 20 minutes.
2. Add tomato juice; cover and cook gently for 10 minutes or until the beef and vegetables are properly cooked. Remove bay leaves.

3. Homemade Creamy Tomato Soup.

Ingredients:-

- 1 tin can (29 oz.) tomato sauce
- 1 cup heavy whipping cream
- 1-1/2 tsp. brown sugar
- 1 tsp. Italian seasoning
- 1/4 tsp. salt to taste
- 1/8 tsp. white pepper
- Warm pepper sauce
- Salad croutons, finely chopped cheddar cheese, quartered grape tomatoes and chopped green onions

Instructions:-

1. In a large skillet, combine the first 7 ingredients. Cook and mix over low heat until heated completely (do not boil). Garnish with croutons, tomatoes, onions and cheese.

4. Marvelous Mushroom Soup.

Ingredients:-

- 3 medium onions, thinly sliced
- 2 garlic cloves, shredded
- 1/4 cup butter
- 2 pounds fresh mushrooms, thinly sliced
- 2 cups heavy whipping cream
- 2 cups beef broth
- 1/2 tsp. salt to taste
- 1/2 tsp. pepper
- Fresh parsley, minced and grated parmesan cheese

Instructions:-

1. Cook onions and garlic in butter in a large skillet over medium-low heat and cook gently. Turn down heat to low and add the thinly sliced mushrooms. Cook for 8-10 minutes. Stir seldom.
2. Add the cream, salt, pepper and broth; cook and stir over low heat until heated completely. Garnish with parsley and Parmesan cheese.

5. Smooth Carrot Soup.

Ingredients:-

- 2 cups thinly sliced carrots
- 1/4 cup thinly sliced onion
- 1 tsp. butter
- 1 tin can (14-1/2 oz.) chicken broth
- 1/4 tsp. fresh ground ginger
- 1/2 cup buttermilk

Instructions:-

1. Fry carrots and onions in butter in a large skillet until crisp-tender. Add broth and ginger. Bring to boil. Turn down heat; cover and cook gently for 10-15 minutes or until carrots are properly cooked. Cool moderately.
2. Blend soup in the blender, return to the skillet. Mix in buttermilk; heat properly (do not boil).

6. Reuben Soup.

Ingredients:-

- 1/2 cup thinly sliced onion
- 1/2 cup chopped celery
- 2 tbsp. butter
- 1 cup chicken broth
- 1/2 tsp. baking soda
- 2 tbsp. cornstarch
- 2 tbsp. water
- 3/4 cup sauerkraut, washed and drained
- 2 cups half-and-half cream
- 2 cups sliced cooked corned beef
- 1 cup (4 oz.) minced Swiss cheese
- Fresh pepper and salt according to taste

Instructions:-

1. Take a large skillet, fry onion and celery properly in butter. Mix broth and baking soda. Mix cornstarch and water until smooth; slowly add to pan. Bring to boil; cook properly and stir for 2 minutes.
2. Turn down heat. Mix sauerkraut, corned beef and cream; cook gently and stir for 15 minutes. Mix cheese and heat until cheese is melted. Add fresh pepper and Salt to taste.

7. Cream of Cauliflower Soup.

Ingredients:-

- 1/3 cups green onions (tops only)
- 2 tbsp. butter
- 2 tbsp. all-purpose flour
- 1/2 tsp. salt
- 2 cups chicken broth
- 2-1/4 cups fresh chilled cauliflower, defrosted and sliced
- 2 cups 1% milk
- 1-1/2 cup (6 oz.) minced low-fat cheddar cheese
- 2 tbsp. dry sherry, optional
- 1 tbsp. shredded chives

Instructions:-

1. In a large skillet, fry onions in butter properly. Mix properly flour and salt together. Slowly add broth. Bring to boil; cook and mix for two minutes. Slow down heat.
2. Add cauliflower, cook gently about two minutes. Add milk and cheese then cook and stir until cheese is melted. Stir in sherry. Garnish with chives.

Snacks:-

1. Chocolate pro Cake.

Ingredients:-

- 4 spoons of chocolate protein powder
- 1 cup chocolate almond oil, unsweetened
- 1.5 ounce dark chocolate
- 2 cups egg whites
- 1/2 tsp. baking powder
- 4 tsp. sucralose based sweetener
- 4 tbsp. cocoa powder, unsweetened

Instructions:-

1. Mix all ingredients.
2. Stir and put in the cake pan.
3. Bake at 190 degree C for 25 minutes or until fully cooked.

2. Mini Cheeseburger Pies.

Ingredients:-

- 1 tbsp. Worcestershire sauce
- 1/2 cup original mix of Bisquick
- 6 tbsp. egg whites
- 1/2 tsp. garlic salt to taste
- 1 cup Colby jack cheese, finely chopped
- 1/2 cup 1 % fat milk
- 1 pound ground beef

Instructions:-

1. Turn on oven to 190 °C. Apply cooking spray to 12 regular size muffin cups.
2. Cook beef over medium heat for 7-8 minutes in a large frying pan, stirring regularly, until cooked properly. Once done, filter and cool for 5 minutes.
3. Add cheese and garlic salt in Worcestershire sauce.
4. Add egg whites, milk and Bisquick, mix well in a medium bowl.
5. In each muffin cup, scoop 1 tbsp. Bisquick mixture and topping with 1/4 cup burger mixture.
6. Bake on low settings for 30 minutes or until cooked fully and muffins are golden brown and cool for 5 minutes.
7. Take out muffins from pan with a thin knife. Put on cooling rack, cool for 10 more minutes.
8. Enjoy your Mini Cheeseburger Pies.

3. Spinach Loaf.

Ingredients:-

- 1 tbsp. butter
- 1 tsp. fresh garlic, shredded
- 1 tbsp. sea salt
- 12 large whole eggs, beaten
- 1 tsp. black pepper to taste
- 30 ounces frozen spinach

Instructions:-

1. Heat up oven to 350 175 °C. Butter loaf pan.
2. Combine garlic, eggs and spinach.
3. Add pepper and sea salt to taste.
4. Pour the mixture over loaf pan and bake for approx. 70 minutes.
5. When done, cool for 12-15 minutes. Take out from loaf pan and cut into slices.
6. Enjoy your yummy Spinach loaf.

4. Cheese Spread.

Ingredients:-

- 5.3 ounces Greek yogurt
- 1 cup cream cheese and Greek yogurt
- 2 cups cheddar cheese, finely minced
- 4 tsp. fresh mix seasoning

Instructions:-

1. Combine all of the ingredients together.
2. Enjoy with celery or crackers.

5. Spinach Egg Muffins.

Ingredients:-

- 6 large Eggs
- 2 ounces sharp cheddar cheese
- 1 cup 2% milk
- 3 medium mushrooms, thinly sliced
- 1 medium onion, finely sliced
- 1 cup fresh spinach

Instructions:-

1. Heat up oven to 175 °C.
2. Take two bowls, beat eggs and milk separately. Mix spices like paprika, black pepper, garlic salt and turmeric.
3. Cut the mushrooms, spinach and onions finely and fry the onions.
4. Apply baking spray on muffin pan. Fill each cavity about half way with spinach, onions and mushrooms evenly. Transfer egg batter about 3/4 of the way into each cavity.
5. Bake approx. 15 minutes then top with cheese and again bake for a further 7-8 minutes.
6. Enjoy your yummy dish.

6. Herbed Tortilla Chips.

Ingredients:-

- 2 tsp. Parmesan Cheese, chopped
- 1/2 tsp. Oregano, dried
- 1/2 tsp. parsley flakes, dried
- 1/2 tsp. rosemary, dried and crumpled
- 1/4 tsp. garlic powder
- 1/8 tsp. Kosher salt to taste
- Small Pinch of Pepper
- 2 flour tortillas
- 2 tsp. olive oil

Instructions:-

1. Mix the first 7 ingredients in a small bowl, sliced each tortillas into 6 wedges and coat with oil. Apply a single layer of cooking spray on baking sheet.
2. Drizzle seasoning mixture on the wedges and bake at 220 degree C for approx. 6-8 minutes or until the color changes to brown. When done, cool for 5 minutes.
3. Enjoy your Herbed Tortilla Chips.

7. Tuna Bites.

Ingredients:-

- 1/4 tsp. garlic salt to taste
- 1/2 tsp. fresh herb mix
- 2 tsp. olive oil
- 1 Egg
- 2 tin cans tuna
- 2 oz. gouda cheese
- 3 tbsp. fresh onion, chopped
- 1/2 fresh spinach

Instructions:-

1. Fry the onion in olive oil with spices and garlic salt, place aside when fried well.
2. Chopped the cheese. Take a large bowl and mix all the ingredients including fried onions, properly.
3. Brush the cooking pan with non-stick spray, put the mixture in 12 equal parts on it.
4. Once completed, cook for 10 minutes, Cook the cake on both side evenly or until the color changes to brown.

8. Egg Muffins with Turkey Sausage.

Ingredients:-

- 12 lean turkey breakfast sausage links
- 12 Eggs
- 5 ounce fresh spinach
- 15 fresh long sweet potato

Instructions:-

1. Beat the eggs in the large bowl and keep aside.
2. Cook sausage properly, slice sweet potato and fry with spinach.
3. Mix cooked sausage, spinach, sweet potato, salt and pepper to bowl with beaten eggs and mix properly.
4. Place mixture into coated muffin pan and filling 3/4 part of the cups. Cook the eggs completely for 20 minutes.
5. Enjoy yummy Egg Muffins with Turkey sausage.
6.

Thank you so much dear reader. I hope you will love all my low carb recipes and will lose weight fast while remain healthy. So just enjoy your food with low carb recipes and get into shape.

Please review this book after reading so that we make changes according to your point of view.

PLEASE ALWAYS KEEP IN TOUCH WITH ME TO UPDATE YOURSELF WITH MY BOOKS.

EMAIL Athar Husain at--atharhusain2015@gmail.com

Also by- Athar Husain:

50 Incredibly delicious low carb recipes for fast and healthy Weight loss!

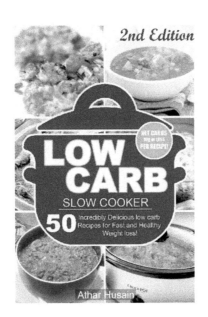